# The Ultimate Pescatarian Cookbook

*Easy and Tasty Recipes for Weight Loss and a Healthy Lifestyle*

Jacob Aiello

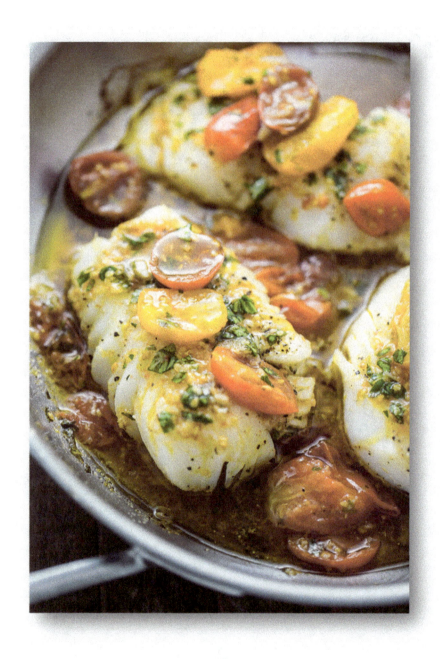

© copyright 2021 – all rights reserved.

the content contained within this book may not be reproduced, duplicated or transmitted without direct written permission from the author or the publisher.

under no circumstances will any blame or legal responsibility be held against the publisher, or author, for any damages, reparation, or monetary loss due to the information contained within this book. either directly or indirectly.

legal notice:

this book is copyright protected. this book is only for personal use. you cannot amend, distribute, sell, use, quote or paraphrase any part, or the content within this book, without the consent of the author or publisher.

disclaimer notice:

please note the information contained within this document is for educational and entertainment purposes only. all effort has been executed to present accurate, up to date, and reliable, complete information. no warranties of any kind are declared or implied. readers acknowledge that the author is not engaging in the rendering of legal, financial, medical or professional advice. the content within this book has been derived from various sources. please consult a licensed professional before attempting any techniques outlined in this book.

by reading this document, the reader agrees that under no circumstances is the author responsible for any losses, direct or indirect, which are incurred as a result of the use of information contained within this document, including, but not limited to, — errors, omissions, or inaccuracies.

# Table of Contents

KETO SEAFOOD CHOWDER ............................................................... 6
20 MINUTES FISH STEW ................................................................... 8
BLACKENED TILAPIA TACOS ............................................................ 10
LOW CARB FLAXSEED TORTILLAS ..................................................... 13
LOW CARB KETO FISH AND CHIPS (GLUTEN FREE) ............................. 16
LOW CARB TUNA ROLLS ................................................................. 19
LEMON DILL TUNA CAKES .............................................................. 21
TUNA STUFFED AVOCADOS ............................................................ 23
CRAB STUFFED AVOCADO WITH LIME ............................................. 25
KETO FRIED SHRIMP ...................................................................... 27
CRISPY COD WITH KETO CHEESE SAUCE AND BROCCOLI ................. 30
TUSCAN BUTTER SALMON ............................................................. 33
LEMON GARLIC SHRIMP ................................................................. 36
KETO BAKED SALMON ................................................................... 38
GARLIC SHRIMP ZOODLES ............................................................. 40
KETO CRAB CAKES (GLUTEN-FREE) ................................................ 42
LOW CARB TUNA SALAD ............................................................... 44

## VEGETARIAN MAIN DISHES ............................................................ 47

CANNELLINI BEANS WITH EGGPLANT ............................................. 47
RED LENTIL FRITTERS .................................................................... 49
FETA OMELETTE ........................................................................... 51
PUMPKIN PASTRY ......................................................................... 53
BAKED APPLES ............................................................................. 55
BULGARIAN BAKED BEANS ........................................................... 56
RICE STUFFED BELL PEPPERS ........................................................ 58
BEANS STUFFED BELL PEPPERS ..................................................... 60
MONASTERY STEW ....................................................................... 62
RICE WITH SPINACH ...................................................................... 64
EGGPLANT AND CHICKPEA STEW .................................................. 66
TURKISH GREEN BEANS ................................................................ 68

Rice and Cabbage Stew ............................................................................. 70

## VEGETARIAN SOUPS ......................................................................... 72

Roasted Red Pepper Soup ...................................................................... 72
Vegetarian Gazpacho .............................................................................. 74
Creamy Zucchini Soup ............................................................................ 76
Celery Root Soup ..................................................................................... 78
Moroccan Lentil Soup ............................................................................. 80
Delicious Minestrone Soup .................................................................... 82
Beet and Carrot Soup .............................................................................. 84
Green Lentil Soup with Rice .................................................................. 86
Broccoli and Potato Soup ....................................................................... 88
Tomato Soup with Rice ........................................................................... 90
Chickpea and Carrot Soup ..................................................................... 92
Spiced Carrot Soup .................................................................................. 94
Mushroom, Barley and Lentil Soup ...................................................... 96
Creamy Wild Mushroom Soup .............................................................. 98

## VEGETARIAN SALADS ...................................................................... 99

Mediterranean Buckwheat Salad .......................................................... 99
Beet and Bean Sprout Salad ................................................................. 101
Tasty Tabbouleh ..................................................................................... 102
Savory Fatoush ....................................................................................... 104
Chickpea Salad (Greek Style) ............................................................... 106
Red Cabbage Salad ................................................................................ 108

# *Keto Seafood Chowder*

**Servings:** 4

**Total Time:** 40 Minutes

## Ingredients and Quantity

- 4 tbsp. almond butter
- 2 garlic cloves, minced
- 1 1/2 cups (5 oz.) celery stalks, sliced
- 1 cup clam juice
- 1 1/2 coconut cream
- 2 tsp. dried sage or dried thyme
- 1/2 lemon, juice and zest
- 4 oz. vegan cheese
- 1 lb. salmon or boneless fillets, cut into 1 inch pieces
- 2 cups (2 oz.) baby spinach
- 8 oz. shrimp peeled and deveined
- Salt and ground black pepper
- 1/2 tbsp. red chili peppers
- Fresh sage, optional, for garnishing

## Direction

1. Melt almond butter in a large pot over medium heat.
2. Add garlic and celery. Cook for about 5 minutes, stirring occasionally. Add clam juice, coconut cream, vegan cheese, sage, lemon juice and lemon zest. Let it simmer for about 10 minutes without lid.
3. Add the fish and shrimp. Simmer for 3 minutes or until fish is just cooked. Add the baby spinach and stir and until wilted.
4. Season with salt and pepper, to taste.
5. Garnish with fresh red chili and fresh sage before serving for extra flavor and splash of color. Enjoy!

# *20 Minutes Fish Stew*

**Servings:** 4

**Total Time:** 23 Minutes

**Ingredients and Quantity:**

- 2 tbsp. olive oil
- 1 small white onion
- 2 cloves garlic, minced
- 1 1/2 lb. wild cod
- 15 oz. can diced tomato
- 1/2 cup coconut milk
- 1/4 cup coconut cream, optional
- 2 tbsp. tomato paste
- 1 whole red, green and yellow bell pepper, sliced in rounds
- 1 pinch sea salt and ground black pepper
- 1/2 tsp. red pepper flakes
- 1 tbsp. fresh cilantro

**Direction**

1. Heat oil in a large skillet or cast iron. Add onion and garlic, cook until fragrant, about 3 minutes.
2. Now add diced tomatoes and stir. Add coconut milk, sour cream (optional) and tomato paste. Stir the sauce and allow to cook for about 3 minutes.
3. Add the sliced pepper and cod chunks. Then season with salt, pepper and red pepper flakes.
4. Cover and allow the fish to simmer for about 10 to 12 minutes. When the fish has cooked for about 7 to 8 minutes, carefully turn the cod so that the other side will be properly cooked in the broth.
5. When done, garnish with fresh cilantro. Serve and enjoy!

# *Blackened Tilapia Tacos*

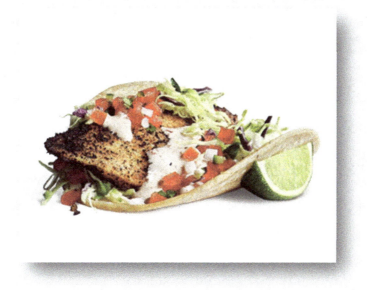

**Servings:** 4

**Total Time:** 23 Minutes

**Calories:** 266

**Fat:** 18.9 g

**Protein:** 14 g

**Carbs:** 3.5 g

**Fiber:** 3 g

## Ingredients and Quantity

### For the Blackened Tilapia:

- 1/2 pound tilapia
- 1 tsp. chili powder
- 1 tsp. paprika
- Salt and pepper, to taste

### For the Cabbage Slaw:

- 1/2 cup red cabbage
- 1 tbsp. olive oil
- 1 tbsp. lime juice
- 1 tsp. apple cider vinegar

### For the Tortillas:

- 1/2 cup flaxseed meal
- 1 tbsp. psyllium husk powder
- 1/2 cup plus 1 tbsp. water
- 2 tbsp. olive oil
- 4 tbsp. guacamole
- Spices of your choice

## Direction

1. Make a half batch of flax seed tortillas.
2. Thinly chop about 1/2 cup red cabbage.
3. Use 1 tablespoon olive oil, juice of 1 lime (about 1 tablespoon) and 1 teaspoon apple cider vinegar to dress the cabbage. Mix well and set aside.
4. Use chili powder, paprika, salt and pepper to season both sides of the tilapia.
5. Add 1 tbsp. olive oil in a sauce pan and heat it up in medium heat.
6. Add the fish and cook each side for about 3 minutes. Make sure the outside is a bit blackened, but not burnt
7. Remove the fish from the pan and set aside for some time.
8. Assemble tacos by placing fish, red cabbage, guacamole and sour cream (1 tablespoon per taco). Squeeze fresh lime juice on top. Then add a bit of cilantro. Serve and enjoy!

# *Low Carb Flaxseed Tortillas*

**Servings:** 4

**Total Time:** 30 Minutes

**Calories:** 184.4

**Fat:** 11.8 g

**Protein:** 5 g

**Carbs:** 2.2 g

**Fiber:** 2.4 g

**Ingredients and Quantity**

- 1 cup golden flaxseed meal
- 2 tbsp. phyllium husk powder
- 2 tsp. olive oil
- 1/4 tsp. xanthan gum
- 1/2 tsp. curry powder
- 1 cup plus 2 tbsp. filtered water

**Per tortilla:** 1 tsp. olive oil, for frying and 1/2 tsp. coconut flour for rolling.

**Direction**

1. In a mixing bowl, add 1 cup golden flaxseed meal, 2 tbsp. psyllium husk powder, 1/4 tsp. xanthan Gum and 1/2 tsp. curry powder or spices of your choice.
2. Mix all of the dry ingredients together well.
3. Now add 2 tsp. olive oil and 1 cup plus 2 tbsp. filtered water to the mixture. Mix well until a solid ball is formed out of the mixture.
4. Leave this ball uncovered on the countertop so that all liquid will be absorbed by the flax meal.
5. Next, measure out portions of tortillas and get a silpat ready. If using a tortilla press, measure out 5 portions. If you are rolling by hand, measure 3 to 4 portions out.
6. For each portion, press it against the silpat with your hands.
7. Sprinkle about 1/2 tsp. coconut flour over the tortilla and rolling pin. Roll out the dough as flat as you can without tearing it.
8. Using a large round object (I used the lid of a pan), cut out your tortilla and separate it from the excess dough. You can use the excess dough to roll out more tortillas.
9. You will have a perfectly round tortilla. Repeat this process for each tortilla.

10. Place a pan over medium-high heat and add 1 tsp. olive oil.
11. Add the tortilla and fry until brown once the oil is hot.
12. You can add fillings of your choice. Serve and enjoy!

# Low Carb Keto Fish and Chips (Gluten Free)

**Servings:** 2

**Total Time:** 45 Minutes + 2 Hours Marinating Time

**Calories:** 242

**Fat:** 13 g

**Protein:** 26 g

**Carbs:** 1 g

**Fiber:** 1 g

**Ingredients and Quantity**

**For the Keto Fish Tacos:**

- 250 g firm white-flesh fish, preferably cod 1/3 cup coconut cream
- 2 tsp. apple cider vinegar
- 4 cloves garlic, ran through a press
- Kosher salt, to taste
- 1/2 cup whey protein isolate

- 1 tsp. baking powder
- 1/4 tsp. garlic powder
- 1/4 to 1/2 tsp. kosher salt, to taste
- 3 tbsp. apple sauce
- 2 tsp. apple cider vinegar
- Coconut oil, or any other healthy cooking oil of your choice

**Optional Serving Suggestions:**

1 batch jicama fries, 8 tortillas

1 batch vegan keto mayonnaise

Lemon

Vinegar

**Direction**

1. Mix the coconut cream, vinegar and garlic. Season to taste with salt.
2. Cut the fish across the grain of the flesh into stripes roundly, 2 inches wide and add them to the cream marinade.
3. Cover and refrigerate for 2 hours.
4. Optionally you can make a batch of keto jicama fries.

5. Add enough oil to a skillet or frying pan to make it about 1/2 inch deep. Use a narrower pan to save a lot of oil. Then heat up the oil over medium-low heat while coating the fish.
6. In a shallow dish, mix the whey protein, baking powder, garlic powder and salt.
7. In a second plate, mix the apple sauce and the vinegar.
8. Dip the fish in the apple sauce mix and then in the whey protein mix. Make sure these mixtures coat the fish properly.
9. Now place the coated fish in the hot oil and blast the top immediately.
10. Fry both sides until deep golden. Then transfer to a paper-lined plate for some minutes.
11. Serve immediately, together with the jicama fries, enough lemon, vegan keto mayo and a drizzle of vinegar. Enjoy!

# Low Carb Tuna Rolls

**Servings:** 3

**Total Time:** 30 Minutes

## Ingredients and Quantity

- 1 medium sized cucumber
- 1 can or pouch of tuna
- 1 tbsp. vegan mayo
- 2 tsp. sriracha
- 2 tsp. garlic powder
- Salt and pepper, to taste
- Avocado, sliced and cut to match the width of cucumber strips

## For the Sauce:

- 2 tbsp. vegan mayo
- 2 tsp. Sriracha

## Direction

1. Use a vegetable peeler to slice the cucumber lengthwise in order to get thin strips.
2. Drain the tuna if necessary and mix with the vegan mayo, sriracha, garlic powder, salt and pepper. Ensure that the mixture is a bit moist, but not too wet.
3. Now place the cucumber strips on prep surface and neatly spread tuna mixture tightly along leaving about 1 inch at the end of the strip.
4. Next, place avocado pieces at end of cucumber strip on top of tuna and roll tightly.
5. For the sauce, mix the vegan mayo and sriracha. Then drizzle over cucumber rolls. Serve and enjoy!

# Lemon Dill Tuna Cakes

**Servings:** 8

**Total Time:** 20 Minutes

**Calories:** 215

**Fat:** 14.2 g

**Protein:** 22.2 g

**Carbs:** 1.7 g

**Fiber:** 0.7 g

## Ingredients and Quantity

- 4 (5 oz.) cans tuna, drained
- 1/3 cup almond flour
- 3 medium green onions, chopped, white and light green parts only
- 2 tbsp. chopped fresh dill
- 1 tbsp. lemon zest
- 3/4 tsp. Salt
- 1/2 tsp. Pepper
- 1/4 cup vegan mayo

- 3 tbsp. apple sauce
- 1 tbsp. freshly squeezed lemon juice
- 2 tbsp. avocado oil

**Direction**

1. Mix together all the ingredients all other ingredients in a large bowl, except the avocado oil. Mix until well combined.
2. Form 8 patties from the mixture, about 3/4 inch thick.
3. Heat 1 tbsp. avocado oil in a large skillet over medium heat until shimmering. Then add half of the tuna patties. Cook for about 3 to 4 minutes, or until golden brown on the bottom
4. Flip the patties over carefully and cook the other side for another 3 to 4 minutes.
5. Transfer to a paper towel-lined plate. Repeat for the remaining oil and patties.
6. Now top the patties with vegan mayo, lemon and capers (optional). Serve and enjoy!

# *Tuna Stuffed Avocados*

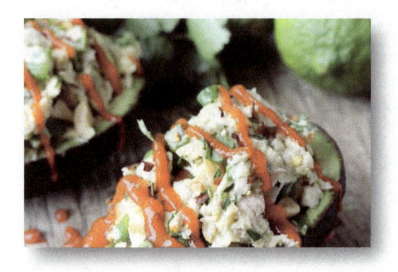

**Servings:** 4

**Total Time:** 15 Minutes

**Calories:** 478

**Fat:** 39 g

**Protein:** 23.3 g

**Carbs:** 12.8 g

**Fiber:** 9.6 g

**Ingredients and Quantity**

- 4 medium size avocados
- 2 (5 oz.) cans tuna
- 1/4 cup vegan mayo
- 1 celery stalk, diced
- 2 tbsp. red onion, diced
- 1/2 tbsp. chopped parsley, chives and other herbs of your choice
- 1/2 tbsp. Dijon mustard
- Salt and pepper, to taste

**Direction**

1. In a mixing bowl, add the tuna, mayonnaise, diced celery, diced red onion, herbs, Dijon mustard, salt and pepper. Stir together until well combined.
2. Slice the avocados in half and remove the seed.
3. Add a few spoonsful of tuna salad onto each avocado half. Serve and enjoy!

# Crab Stuffed Avocado with Lime

**Servings:** 2

**Total Time:** 10 Minutes

**Calories:** 434

**Fat:** 36 g

**Protein:** 11 g

**Carbs:** 12 g

**Fiber:** 10 g

**Ingredients and Quantity**

- 1 ripe California avocado, halved and pitted
- 1/4 cup avocado oil mayonnaise
- 3 tbsp. plus 1 tsp. fresh lime juice, divided
- 2 tbsp. diced onion
- 2 tbsp. chopped fresh cilantro
- 1/2 tsp. ground cumin
- 1/4 tsp. fine sea salt

- Ground pepper, to taste
- 1 (6 oz.) can crab meat (I used lump crab meat)
- Lime wedges, for serving
- Dash sriracha, optional

## Direction

1. Combine the mayonnaise, 3 tbsp. lime juice, onions, cilantro, cumin, salt and pepper in a medium bowl. Gently fold in the crabmeat. Adjust seasoning to taste.
2. Use the remaining lime juice to brush the avocado, to avoid browning.
3. Place avocado halves, cut side up, on plates. Add the crab salad into each avocado half.
4. Serve with lime wedges and dash of sriracha, if desired. Enjoy!

# Keto Fried Shrimp

**Servings:** 8

**Total Time:** 30 Minutes

**Calories:** 475

**Fat:** 37 g

**Protein:** 30.5 g

**Carbs:** 4.8 g

**Fiber:** 2.3 g

## Ingredients and Quantity

### For the Shrimp:

- 350 g peeled raw shrimp (12.4 oz.)
- 1/2 tsp. Dijon mustard
- 1 1/2 tsp. paprika
- 1/2 tsp. thyme
- 1 tsp. garlic powder
- 1/2 tsp. cayenne pepper
- 1 tsp. dried oregano
- 3/4 cup whey protein powder

- 5 tbsp. apple sauce
- 1 tbsp. coconut cream
- 1/2 tsp. hot sauce, or to taste
- 1 tsp. flaked sea salt
- 1/4 tsp. cracked black pepper
- 2 cups avocado or coconut oil, for frying

**For the Slaw:**

- 2 cups shredded white cabbage
- 1 cup shredded red cabbage
- 1 medium celery, sliced
- 1 medium spring onion, sliced
- 2 tbsp. vegan mayo
- 1 tsp. lemon juice
- Pinch sea salt

**Direction**

1. In a bowl, mix the dry ingredients: paprika, thyme, garlic powder, cayenne pepper, oregano, pinch of salt and whey protein powder.
2. In another bowl, mix the wet ingredients: apple sauce, coconut cream, hot sauce, Dijon mustard and a pinch of salt.

3. Dip the shrimp in the wet mixed ingredients and then in the dry ingredients. Shake off the excess ingredients. Do this in small batches of 5 shrimps at a time to avoid clumping.
4. Add the avocado or coconut oil to a deep pan (about 7.5 inches) that will allow the shrimp to be completely submerged.
5. Heat up the oil and then fry the shrimp on a medium-low heat for about 1 to 2 minutes or until golden and cooked through. Do the frying in batches of 5 shrimps at a time for even frying and no clumping.
6. Use a slotted spoon to drain the shrimp from the oil. Use a paper towel to absorb excess oil while frying the other batches.
7. For the slaw, simply mix all the ingredients together in a bowl.
8. Serve the fried shrimp with the slaw. Optionally, you can serve with a vegan mayo. Enjoy!

# Crispy Cod with Keto Cheese Sauce and Broccoli

**Servings:** 4

**Total Time:** 20 Minutes

**Calories:** 433

**Fat:** 29.3 g

**Protein:** 34.9 g

**Carbs:** 6.4 g

**Fiber:** 2.3 g

## Ingredients and Quantity

### For the Cheese Sauce:

- 2 tbsp. coconut cream
- 1 tbsp. almond butter
- 2 tbsp. vegan cheese
- Pinch sea salt, optional
- 1 tbsp. water, or more if you need to thin it down

**For the Cod and Broccoli:**

- 1 (250 g) small bunch broccoli
- 2 skin-on cod loins (300 g)
- Sea salt and pepper, to taste
- 1 tbsp. avocado oil

**Direction**

1. To make the cheese sauce, place the coconut cream and almond butter into a small sauce pan and gently heat up. Add the vegan cheese.
2. Stir until melted and then bring to a simmer. Once bubbles start forming, remove the heat source.
3. Mix until smooth and creamy. For a thicker sauce, you can cook for extra 3 to 5 minutes while stirring. You can add a splash of water or coconut cream.
4. Pat the cod loins dry with a paper towel. Season both sides with salt and pepper.
5. Pour the avocado oil in a skillet or a non-stick pan and heat up over medium-high heat.
6. Add the cod loins, skin side down. Cook for 3 to 5 minutes, depending on the thickness of the fish, or until the skin is crisped on and the sides are opaque. Flip the fish and cook for another 1 to 2 minutes. When done, set aside and keep warm.

7. Cut the ends off the broccoli and cut in half. Then place the broccoli florets in a double boiler or a pot filled with boiling water. Cook for 4 to 5 minutes, or until the broccoli becomes crisp-tender.
8. Serve the broccoli with the crispy cod and cheese sauce immediately. Sprinkle with more pepper to taste. Enjoy!
9. You can serve immediately or store for up to a day. But you need to reheat gently before eating the next day.

# *Tuscan Butter Salmon*

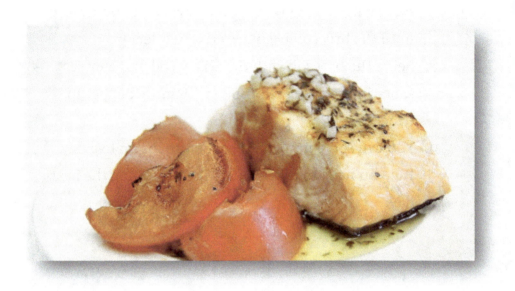

**Servings:** 4

**Total Time:** 45 Minutes

**Ingredients and Quantity**

- 2 tbsp. extra virgin olive oil
- 4 (6 oz.) salmon fillets, patted dry with paper towels
- 3 cloves garlic, minced
- 1 1/2 cups halved cherry tomatoes
- 2 cups baby spinach
- 1/2 cup coconut cream

- 1/4 cup vegan cheese
- 1/4 cup chopped herbs (basil and parsley), plus more for garnishing
- Kosher salt, to taste
- Freshly ground black pepper
- Lemon wedges, for serving (optional)

**Direction**

1. Heat the oil in a large skillet over medium-high heat. Season the salmon all over with salt and pepper.
2. Immediately the oil starts shimmering, add the salmon, skin side up and cook for about 6 minutes or until deep golden. Flip over and cook 2 more minutes. Then transfer to a plate.
3. Reduce the heat to medium and then add the almond butter. Wait for the butter to melt and then stir in the garlic. Cook for 1 minute or until fragrant.
4. Add cherry tomatoes and then season with salt and pepper. Cook until the tomatoes begin to burst.
5. Now add spinach and cook until they begin to wilt.

6. Stir in the heavy cream, vegan cheese and hers. Then bring the mixture to a simmer.
7. Reduce the heat to low and simmer for about 3 minutes or until sauce is slightly reduced.
8. Put back the salmon in a skillet and spoon over sauce. Simmer for about 3 minutes or until salmon is cooked through.
9. Use the herbs to garnish it and squeeze lemon on top before you serve. Enjoy!

# *Lemon Garlic Shrimp*

**Servings:** 4

**Total Time:** 15 Minutes

## Ingredients and Quantity

- 2 tbsp. almond butter, divided
- 1 tbsp. extra-virgin olive oil
- 1 lb. medium shrimp, peeled and deveined
- 1 lemon, thinly sliced, plus juice from 1 lemon
- 3 cloves garlic, minced
- 1 tsp. crushed red pepper flakes
- Kosher salt
- 2 tbsp. dry white wine, or water
- Freshly chopped parsley, for garnishing

**Direction**

1. Melt 1 tablespoon each of almond butter and olive oil in a large skillet over medium heat.
2. Add the shrimp, crushed red pepper flakes, lemon slices, garlic and then season with salt.
3. Cook for about 3 minutes per side or until shrimp turns pink and opaque, stirring occasionally.
4. Remove the skillet containing the shrimp from the heat source and then stir in the remaining almond butter, lemon juice and white wine.
5. Season with salt and garnish with parsley before serving. Enjoy!

# *Keto Baked Salmon*

**Servings:** 4

**Total Time:** 30 Minutes

**Calories:** 303

**Fat:** 19 g

**Protein:** 30 g

**Carbs:** 3 g

**Fiber:** 2 g

**Ingredients and Quantity**

- 1 tsp. avocado oil
- 2 tbsp. soy sauce
- 2 tbsp. rice vinegar
- 4 tsp. sesame oil
- 4 (4 to 5 oz.) salmon fillets
- 1/2 tsp. sea salt
- 1/2 tsp. black pepper
- 1/4 cup sesame seeds
- 2 tsp. fresh thyme

**Direction**

1. Preheat your oven to 400 F.
2. Use a paper towel to pat the salmon dry and then season it with salt and pepper.
3. Use avocado oil to lightly grease a baking dish and then place the salmon fillets in it.
4. Whisk together the soy sauce, rice vinegar and sesame oil in a small bowl.
5. Then pour the mixture over the salmon and bake for about 15 minutes, or until the salmon is fully cooked.
6. Now sprinkle the sesame seeds before serving. You can pair it with cauliflower. Serve and enjoy!

# *Garlic Shrimp Zoodles*

**Servings:** 2

**Total Time:** 15 Minutes

**Calories:** 276

**Fat:** 10 g

**Protein:** 38 g

**Carbs:** 9 g

**Fiber:** 2 g

**Ingredients and Quantity**

- 2 medium zucchini
- 3/4 pounds medium shrimp, peeled and deveined
- 1 tbsp. olive oil
- Juice and zest of 1 lemon
- 3 to 4 cloves garlic, minced
- Salt and pepper, to taste
- Fresh parsley, chopped
- Red pepper flakes, optional

**Direction**

1. Use a spiralizer to spiralize the zucchini on the medium setting. Set aside.
2. In a skillet over medium heat, add the olive oil lemon juice and zest.
3. Once the pan has heat up a bit, add the shrimp and cook for 1 minute per side.
4. Add the garlic and red pepper flakes. Cook for extra 1 minute, stirring continuously.
5. Add the zucchini noodles and toss (with tongs) continuously for about 2 to 3 minutes until they are slightly cooked and warmed up.
6. Season with salt and pepper. Then sprinkle the chopped parsley on top. Serve immediately. Enjoy!

# Keto Crab Cakes (Gluten-Free)

**Servings:** 8

**Total Time:** 30 Minutes

**Calories:** 106

**Fat:** 7 g

**Protein:** 9 g

**Carbs:** 12 g

**Fiber:** 0.4 g

**Ingredients and Quantity**

- 1 lb. lump crab meat
- 1/2 cup onion, finely chopped
- 3 tbsp. blanched almond flour, or golden flaxseed, for nut-free diet
- 1/4 cup apple sauce
- 2 tbsp. Worcestershire sauce
- 1 tsp. mustard
- 1 tbsp. dried parsley

- 1 tbsp. old bay seasoning
- 2 tbsp. olive oil, divided

## Direction

1. In a skillet, heat 2 tbsp. olive oil over medium heat. Then sauté the chopped onion for about 10 minutes, or until translucent and lightly browned.
2. Meanwhile, mix all the other ingredients except the crab meat and the remaining olive oil, until well combined. Then add the sautéed onions. Finally, fold in crab meat very gently. Avoid breaking up the lumps of crab meat.
3. Form 8 patties and then place them on a lined baking sheet or cutting board. You can refrigerate for like 30 minutes so that the crab cakes will stay together when frying.
4. In a skillet over medium heat, fry the crab cakes in two batches. Use about 2 tbsp. olive oil for each batch and cook for about 3 to 5 minutes per side, until browned. Serve and enjoy!

# *Low Carb Tuna Salad*

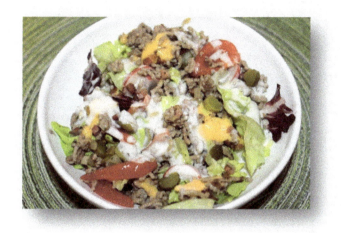

**Servings:** 8

**Total Time:** 10 Minutes

**Calories:** 167

**Ingredients and Quantity**

- 2 (12 oz.) cans tuna, solid white Albacore in water
- 3 to 4 celery stalks, diced (about 1 1/2 cups)
- 1/3 cup shallot, small dice (1 medium shallot can serve)
- 1 1/4 cups avocado oil mayo
- 1 tbsp. celery seed

- 2 tbsp. fresh lemon juice
- 1 tsp. salt

**Direction**

1. Drain the tuna and add to a large bowl.
2. In a medium bowl, add all remaining ingredients and mix well.
3. Adjust the seasonings to your taste. Serve cold. Enjoy!

# VEGETARIAN RECIPES

The vegetarian recipes in this cookbook were inspired by the Mediterranean lifestyle, which helps you cook delicious meals with healthy, locally available ingredients that you can buy or even grow in your backyard. Some of the commonly used ingredients in these vegetarian recipes include: extra virgin olive oil, fresh vegetables, protein-rich legumes, nuts, seeds, healthy cheeses, aromatic, super food herbs and spices.

All Mediterranean vegetarian dishes are generally prepared slowly in an all-in-one pot and are very rarely fried. Another benefit of vegetarian meal is that they usually have low WW food point scores, most of the dishes even have zero point score. This helps you achieve your weight loss set target within the possible shortest period of time. Not only that, you will also enjoy delicious meals while still meeting your healthy lifestyle and weight loss target. The meals in this cookbook will keep you free from digestion problems, excess weight gain, diabetes and also keep you free from heart diseases.

You will find in this cookbook, delicious vegetarian soups and salads recipes that can serve as main meal, side dish or even use it to garnish your seafood dishes.

**VEGETARIAN MAIN DISHES**

# Cannellini Beans with Eggplant

**Servings:** 4

**Ingredients and Quantity**

- 2 medium sized eggplants, peeled and diced
- 1 can cannellini beans, drained
- 1 cup canned tomatoes, drained and diced
- 1 red bell pepper, chopped
- 1 onion, chopped
- 4 garlic cloves, chopped
- 1 bunch parsley, chopped, for serving
- 3 tbsp. extra virgin olive oil
- 1/2 tsp. paprika
- 1 green chili, chopped
- 1 tbsp. dried mint
- Salt and black pepper, to taste
- 1/2 cup finely cut fresh parsley

**Direction**

1. Gently sauté onion, garlic, eggplants in olive oil on medium-high heat for 6 to 7 minutes.
2. Add in paprika and chili pepper and cook for 1 to 2 minutes, stirring.
3. Add the rest of the ingredients.
4. Cover and simmer on low-high heat for 30 minutes.
5. Sprinkle with parsley. Serve and enjoy!

# Red Lentil Fritters

**Servings:** 4

**Ingredients and Quantity**

- 1 cup dry red lentils
- 1/3 cup bulgur
- 3 garlic cloves, crushed
- 5 to 6 spring onions, finely chopped
- 1/2 cup fresh dill, finely cut
- 5 to 6 fresh mint leaves, chopped
- 1 tbsp. tomato paste
- 1 tsp. cumin
- 1 tsp. paprika
- Salt and black pepper, to taste
- 1/2 cup sunflower oil, for frying

**Direction**

1. Boil lentils in 2 cups of water until the water is almost absorbed.
2. Now add in bulgur and salt. Set aside, covered.

3. When lentil mixture has cooled, add all the other ingredients except the sunflower oil. Stir to combine.
4. Heat the sunflower oil in a frying pan.
5. Drop a few scoops of the lentil mixture and fry them on medium heat, making sure they don't touch.
6. Fry them for 3 to 5 minutes or until golden brown.
7. Serve with vegetable salad. Enjoy!

# *Feta Omelette*

**Servings:** 5

**Ingredients and Quantity**

- 1 small onion, finely cut
- 1 green bell pepper, chopped
- 1 red pepper, chopped
- 4 tomatoes, cubed
- 2 garlic cloves, crushed
- 8 eggs
- 10 oz. feta cheese, crumbled
- 4 tbsp. olive oil
- 1/2 bunch parsley
- Black pepper and salt, to taste

**Direction**

1. In a large pan, sauté onion over medium heat, till transparent.
2. Reduce the heat and add bell peppers and garlic.
3. Continue cooking until soft.
4. Add the tomatoes and continue simmering until the mixture is almost dry.
5. Add the cheese and all the eggs.

6. Stir and cook well until well mixed and not too watery.
7. Season with black pepper and remove from heat.
8. Sprinkle with parsley. Serve and enjoy!

# Pumpkin Pastry

**Servings:** 8

**Ingredients and Quantity**

- 14 oz. filo pastry
- 1 cup pumpkin, shredded
- 1 cup walnuts, coarsely chopped
- 1/2 cup sugar
- 6 tbsp. sunflower oil
- 1 tbsp. cinnamon
- 1 tsp. vanilla

**Direction**

1. Grate the pumpkin and steam it until tender.
2. Cool and add the walnuts, sugar, cinnamon and vanilla.
3. Place a few sheets of pastry in the baking dish.
4. Sprinkle with oil and spread the filling on top.
5. Repeat this a few times finishing with a sheet of pastry.
6. Bake for 20 minutes at 350 degrees F.

7. Allow the pumpkin pie to cool down and then dust with the powdered sugar. Serve and enjoy!

# Baked Apples

**Servings:** 4

**Ingredients and Quantity**

- 8 medium sized apples
- 1/3 cup walnuts, crushed
- 3/4 cup sugar
- 3 tbsp. raisins, soaked
- Vanilla and cinnamon, to taste
- 2 oz. butter

**Direction**

1. Peel and carefully hollow the apples.
2. Prepare stuffing by beating butter, 3/4 cup of sugar, crushed walnuts, raisins and cinnamon.
3. Stuff the apples and place in an oiled dish.
4. Pour over 1 to 2 tbsp. of water and bake in a moderate oven.
5. Serve warm with a scoop of vanilla ice cream. Enjoy!

# *Bulgarian Baked Beans*

**Servings:** 6

## Ingredients and Quantity

- 2 cups dried white beans
- 2 medium onions, chopped
- 1 red bell pepper, chopped
- 1 carrot, chopped
- 1/4 cup sunflower oil
- 1 tsp. paprika
- 1 tsp. black pepper
- 1 tbsp. plain flour
- 1/2 bunch fresh parsley and mint
- 1 tsp. salt

## Direction

1. Wash the beans and soak in water overnight.
2. In the morning, discard the water, pour enough cold water to cover the beans.
3. Add one of the onions, peeled and washed but left whole.

4. Cook until the beans are soft but not falling apart.
5. If there is excess water left, drain the beans.
6. Now, chop the other onion and fry it in a frying pan alongside the chopped bell pepper and the carrot.
7. Add paprika, plain flour and the beans.
8. Stir well and pour the mixture in a baking dish along with some parsley, mint and salt.
9. Bake in an oven preheated to 350 degrees F for 20 to 30 minutes.
10. Don't allow the beans to be too dry or too watery.
11. Best served warm. Enjoy!

# *Rice Stuffed Bell Peppers*

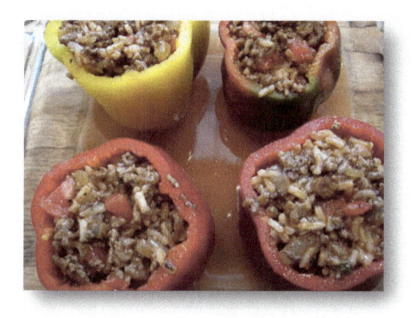

**Servings:** 4

**Ingredients and Quantity**

- 8 bell peppers, cored and seeded
- 1 1/2 cups rice, washed and drained
- 2 onions, chopped
- 1 tomato, chopped
- Fresh parsley, chopped
- 3 tbsp. olive oil
- 1 tbsp. paprika

**Direction**

1. Heat the oil and sauté the onions for 2 to 3 minutes.
2. Add the paprika, the washed and rinsed rice, the tomatoes, and then season with salt and pepper.
3. Add 1/2 cup of hot water and cook the rice until the rice is well cooked and the water is absorbed.
4. Stuff each pepper with the mixture using a spoon. Every pepper should be 3/4 full.
5. Arrange the peppers in a deep ovenproof dish and top up with warm water to half fill the dish.
6. Cover and bake for about 20 minutes at 350 degrees F.
7. Uncover and cook for another 15 minutes until the peppers are well cooked.
8. Serve alone or with plain yogurt.

# Beans Stuffed Bell Peppers

**Servings:** 5

**Ingredients and Quantity**

- 10 dried bell peppers
- 1 cup dried beans
- 1 onion
- 3 garlic cloves
- 2 tbsp. flour
- 1 carrot
- 1 bunch parsley
- 1/2 crushed walnuts
- Some paprika, to taste
- Salt, to taste

**Direction**

1. Put the dried peppers in warm water and leave them there for 1 hour.
2. Now cook the beans.
3. Chop the carrot and the onion, sauté them and add them to the cooked beans.

4. Add as well the finely chopped parsley and the walnuts.
5. Stir the mixture to make it homogeneous.
6. Drain the peppers, then fill them with the mixture and place in a roasting tin.
7. Cover the pepper's openings with flour to seal them during the baking.
8. Bake them for 30 minutes at 350 degrees F. Serve and enjoy!

# *Monastery Stew*

**Servings:** 4

**Ingredients and Quantity**

- 3 to 4 potatoes, diced
- 2 to 3 tomatoes, diced
- 1 to 2 carrots, chopped
- 1 to 2 onions, finely chopped
- 1 cup small shallots, whole
- 1 celery rib, chopped
- 2 cups fresh mushrooms, chopped
- 1/2 cup black olives, pitted
- 1/4 cup rice
- 1/2 cup white wine
- 1/2 cup sunflower oil
- 1 bunch parsley
- 1 tsp. black pepper
- 1 tsp. salt

**Direction**

1. Sauté the finely chopped onions, carrots and celery in a little oil.
2. Add the small onions, olives, mushrooms and black pepper and then stir well.
3. Pour over the wine and 1 cup of water, salt to your taste.
4. Cover and allow to simmer until tender.
5. After 15 minutes, add the diced potatoes, the rice and the tomato pieces.
6. Transfer everything into a clay pot, sprinkle with parsley and bake for about 30 minutes at 350 degrees F. Serve and enjoy!

# Rice with Spinach

**Servings:** 4

## Ingredients and Quantity

- 3 to 4 cups fresh spinach, washed, drained and chopped
- 1/2 cup rice
- 1 onion, chopped
- 1 carrot, chopped
- 1/4 cup extra virgin olive oil
- 2 cups water

## Direction

1. Heat the oil in a large skillet and cook the onions and the carrots until soft.
2. Add the paprika and the washed, rinsed and drained rice and then mix well.
3. Add 2 cups of warm water, stirring constantly as the rice absorbs it.
4. Simmer for more 20 minutes.
5. Wash the spinach well and cut in strips.

6. Add the rice and cook until it wilts.
7. Remove from the heat and season to taste. Serve with yogurt. Enjoy!

# *Eggplant and Chickpea Stew*

**Servings:** 4

**Ingredients and Quantity**

- 2 to 3 eggplants, peeled and diced
- 1 onion, chopped
- 2 to 3 garlic cloves, crushed
- 1 can (15 oz.) chickpeas, drained
- 1 can (15 oz.) tomatoes, undrained, diced
- 1 tsp. paprika
- 1/2 tsp. cinnamon
- 1 tsp. cumin
- 1 tbsp. olive oil
- Salt and pepper, to taste

**Direction**

1. Peel and dice the eggplants.
2. Heat olive oil in a large deep frying pan and sauté onions and crushed garlic.
3. Add paprika, cumin and cinnamon. Stir well to coat evenly.

4. Sauté for 3 to 4 minutes until the onions are soft.
5. Add the eggplant, tomatoes and chickpeas.
6. Bring to a boil, lower the heat and simmer for 10 minutes, covered or until the eggplant is tender.
7. Uncover the simmer for a few more minutes until the liquid evaporates. Serve and enjoy!

# *Turkish Green Beans*

**Servings:** 4

**Ingredients and Quantity**

- 1 lb. green beans, fresh or frozen
- 1 onion, chopped
- 4 garlic cloves, crushed
- 2 large tomatoes, diced
- 1/4 cup sunflower oil
- 1/2 cup hot water
- 1 tbsp. paprika
- 1/4 tsp. cumin
- 1 tsp. salt
- 1 tsp. sugar
- Black pepper, to taste
- 1 bunch fresh parsley, chopped, for serving

**Direction**

1. Sauté the onions and the garlic lightly in olive oil.
2. Add the green beans and the remaining ingredients.
3. Cover and simmer over medium heat for about an hour or until all vegetables are tender.
4. Check after 30 minutes; add more water if necessary.
5. Sprinkle with fresh parsley. Best served warm. Enjoy!

# *Rice and Cabbage Stew*

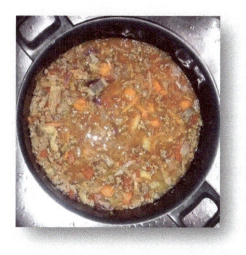

**Servings:** 4

**Ingredients and Quantity**

- 1 cup long grain white rice
- 2 cups water
- 2 tbsp. extra virgin olive oil
- 1 small onion, chopped
- 1 garlic clove, crushed
- 1/4 head cabbage, cored and shredded
- 2 tomatoes, diced
- 1 tbsp. paprika
- 1/2 bunch parsley

- Salt, to taste
- Black pepper, to taste

## Direction

1. Heat the olive oil in a large pot.
2. Add the onion and f=garlic and cook until transparent.
3. Add the paprika, rice and water and then stir and bring to a boil.
4. Simmer for 10 minutes.
5. Add the shredded cabbage, the tomatoes, and cook for about 20 minutes, stirring occasionally until the cabbage cooks down.
6. Season with salt and pepper.
7. Sprinkle with parsley. Serve and enjoy!

**VEGETARIAN SOUPS**

# *Roasted Red Pepper Soup*

**Servings:** 6

## Ingredients and Quantity

- 5 red peppers or more
- 1 large brown onion, chopped
- 2 garlic cloves, crushed
- 4 medium tomatoes, chopped
- 2 cups vegetable broth
- 3 tbsp. olive oil
- 2 bay leaves

## Direction

1. Grill the peppers or roast them in the oven at 400 degrees F until the skins are a little burnt.

2. Place the roasted peppers in a brown paper bag or a lidded container and leave covered for about 10 minutes.

3. This makes it easier to peel them.
4. Peel the skins and remove the seeds.
5. Cut the peppers in small pieces.
6. Heat oil in a large saucepan over medium-high heat.
7. Add onion and garlic and sauté, stirring, for 3 minutes, or until onion has softened.
8. Add the red peppers, bay leaves, tomatoes and simmer for about 5 minutes.
9. Add broth and season with pepper.
10. Bring to boil and then reduce heat and simmer for 20 more minutes.
11. Set aside to cool slightly.
12. Blend in batches, until smooth. Serve and enjoy!

# *Vegetarian Gazpacho*

**Servings:** 6

### Ingredients and Quantity

- 2 1/4 lb. tomatoes, peeled and halved
- 1 onion, sliced
- 1 green pepper, sliced
- 1 big cucumber, peeled and diced
- 2 garlic cloves
- Salt, to taste
- 4 tbsp. olive oil
- 1 tbsp. apple vinegar

### For Garnishing:

- 1/2 onion, chopped
- 1 green pepper, chopped
- 1 cucumber, chopped

**Direction**

1. Place the tomatoes, garlic, onion, green pepper, cucumber, salt, olive oil and vinegar in a blender or food processor and puree until smooth.

2. Add small amount of cold water if necessary to achieve desired consistency.
3. Serve the gazpacho chilled with the chopped onion, green pepper and cucumber. Enjoy!

# *Creamy Zucchini Soup*

**Servings:** 4

**Ingredients and Quantity**

- 1 onion, finely chopped
- 2 garlic cloves, crushed
- 1 cup vegetable broth
- 2 cups water
- 2 zucchinis, peeled, thinly sliced
- 1 big potato, peeled and chopped
- 3 tbsp. olive oil
- 1/4 cup fresh basil leaves
- 1/2 cup yogurt, for serving

**Direction**

1. Heat olive oil in a saucepan over a medium heat.
2. Gently sauté onion and garlic for 1 to 2 minutes.
3. Add in vegetable broth and water and then bring to a boil.
4. Add in the zucchinis, potato and a teaspoon of sugar.

5. Reduce heat to medium-low and simmer, stirring occasionally, for 10 minutes or until the zucchinis are soft.
6. Stir in basil and simmer for 2-3 minutes more.
7. Set aside to cool, then blend in batches and reheat.
8. Serve with a dollop of yogurt and/or sprinkled with Parmesan cheese. Enjoy!

# Celery Root Soup

**Servings:** 4

**Ingredients and Quantity**

- 2 leeks, the white and green parts only, chopped
- 2 garlic cloves, crushed
- 1 large celery root, peeled and diced
- 2 potatoes, peeled and diced
- 4 cups vegetable broth
- 1 bay leaf
- 2 tbsp. extra virgin olive oil
- Salt and black pepper, to taste

**Direction**

1. In a skillet, heat olive oil, then add the leeks and sauté about 3-4 minutes.
2. Add in the garlic and sauté an additional 3-40 seconds.
3. In a slow cooker, add the sautéed leeks and garlic, celeriac, potatoes, broth, bay leaf, salt, and pepper.
4. Cover and cook on low heat for 7-8 hours.

5. Set aside to cool.
6. Now, remove the bay leaf, then process in a blender or with an immersion blender until smooth. Serve and enjoy!

# *Moroccan Lentil Soup*

**Servings:** 10

**Ingredients and Quantity**

- 1 cup red lentils
- 1 cup canned chickpeas, drained
- 2 onions, chopped
- 2 garlic cloves, minced
- 1 cup canned tomatoes, chopped
- 1 cup canned white beans, drained
- 3 carrots, diced
- 3 celery ribs, diced
- 4 cups water
- 3 tbsp. olive oil
- 1 tsp. ginger, grated
- 1 tsp. ground cardamom
- 1/2 tsp. ground cumin

**Direction**

1. In a large pot, sauté onions, garlic and ginger in olive oil for about 5 minutes.
2. Add the water, lentils, chickpeas, white beans, tomatoes, carrots, celery, cardamom and cumin.
3. Bring to a boil for a few minutes, then simmer for half an hour or longer until the lentils are tender.
4. Puree half the soup in a food processor or blender.
5. Return the pureed soup to the pot, stir and serve. Enjoy!

# *Delicious Minestrone Soup*

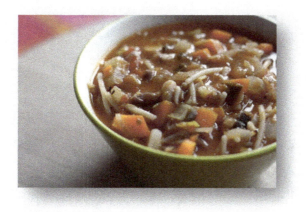

**Servings:** 6

**Ingredients and Quantity**

- 1/4 cabbage, chopped
- 2 carrots, chopped
- 1 celery rib, thinly sliced
- 1 small onion, chopped
- 2 garlic cloves, chopped
- 2 cups water
- 1 cup canned tomatoes, diced, undrained
- 1 cup fresh spinach, torn
- 1/2 cup pasta, cooked

- 2 tbsp. extra virgin olive oil
- Black pepper and salt, to taste

## Direction

1. Sauté the carrots, cabbage, celery, onion and garlic in oil for 5 minutes in a deep saucepan.
2. Add water, tomatoes and bring to a boil.
4. Reduce heat and simmer uncovered, for 20 minutes or until vegetables are tender.
5. Stir in spinach, macaroni, and season with salt and pepper to your taste. Serve and enjoy!

# Beet and Carrot Soup

**Servings:** 6

## Ingredients and Quantity

- 4 beets, washed and peeled
- 2 carrots, peeled, chopped
- 2 potatoes, peeled, chopped
- 1 medium sized onion, chopped
- 2 cups vegetable broth
- 2 cups water
- 2 tbsp. yogurt
- 2 tbsp. olive oil
- 1 bunch of spring onions, cut, for serving

## Direction

1. Peel and chop the beets.
2. Heat olive oil in a saucepan over medium high heat and sauté onion and carrot until onion is tender.
3. Add beets, potatoes, broth and water.
4. Bring to the boil.

5. Reduce heat to medium and simmer, partially covered, for 30-40 minutes, or until beets are tender. Cool slightly.
6. Blend soup in batches until smooth.
7. Return it to pan over low heat and cook, stirring, for 4 to 5 minutes.
8. Serve with soup topped with yogurt and sprinkled with spring onions. Enjoy!

# Green Lentil Soup with Rice

**Servings:** 6

## Ingredients and Quantity

- 1 cup green lentils
- 1 small onion, finely cut
- 1 carrot, chopped
- 5 cups vegetable broth
- 1/4 cup rice
- 1 tbsp. paprika
- Salt and black pepper, to taste
- 1/2 cup finely cut dill, to serve

## Direction

1. Heat oil in a large saucepan and sauté the onion stirring occasionally, until transparent.
2. Add in carrot, paprika and lentils and stir to combine.

3. Add vegetable broth to the saucepan and bring to the boil, then reduce heat and simmer for 20 minutes.
4. Stir in rice and cook on medium low until rice is properly cooked.
5. Sprinkle with dill. Serve and enjoy!

# *Broccoli and Potato Soup*

**Servings:** 6

- **Ingredients and Quantity**
- 2 lb. broccoli, cut into florets
- 2 potatoes, chopped
- 1 big onion, chopped
- 3 garlic cloves, crushed
- 4 cups water
- 1 tbsp. olive oil
- 1/4 tsp. ground nutmeg

**Direction**

1. Heat oil in a large saucepan over medium-high heat.
2. Add onion and garlic and sauté, stirring, for 3 minutes, or until soft.
3. Add broccoli, potato and 4 cups of cold water.
5. Cover and bring to the boil, then reduce heat to low.

6. Simmer, stirring, for 10 to 15 minutes, or until the potatoes are tender.
7. Remove from heat and then blend until smooth.
8. Return to pan. Cook for 5 minutes or until properly cooked. Serve and enjoy!

# *Tomato Soup with Rice*

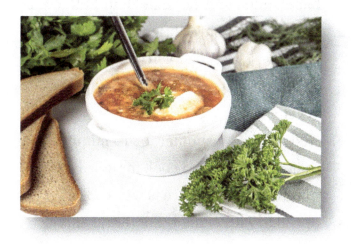

**Servings:** 4

**Ingredients and Quantity**

- 1 large onion, diced
- 1/3 cup rice
- 3 cups water
- 2 garlic cloves, chopped
- 3 tbsp. olive oil
- 1/2 tsp. salt
- ½ tsp. black pepper
- 1 tsp. sugar
- ½ bunch fresh parsley

**Direction**

1. Sauté onion and garlic in oil in a large soup pot.
2. When onions have softened, add tomatoes and cook for 10 minutes.
3. Stir in the spices and sugar and mix well to coat vegetables.
4. Add water and simmer for 10 minutes and then stir in rice and cook for at least 20 minutes or till the rice is well cooked.
5. Sprinkle with parsley. Serve and enjoy!

# Chickpea and Carrot Soup

**Servings:** 4

## Ingredients and Quantity

- 4 big carrots, chopped
- 1 leek, chopped
- 4 cups vegetable broth
- 1 cup canned chickpeas, undrained
- 1/2 cup orange juice
- 2 tbsp. olive oil
- 1/2 tsp. cumin
- 1/2 tsp. ginger
- tbsp. yogurt, for serving

## Direction

1. Heat oil in a large saucepan over medium heat.
2. Add leek and carrots and sauté until soft.
3. Add orange juice, broth, chickpeas and spices.
4. Bring to the boil.
5. Reduce heat to medium-low and simmer, covered, for 15 minutes.

6. Blend soup until smooth; return to pan.
7. Season with salt and pepper. Stir over heat until heated through.
8. Pour in about 4 bowls.
9. Top with yogurt. Serve and enjoy!

# Spiced Carrot Soup

**Servings:** 6

## Ingredients and Quantity

- 10 carrots, peeled and chopped
- 2 medium sized onions, chopped
- 4 cups water or more
- 2 garlic cloves, minced
- 1 big red chili pepper, finely chopped
- 5 tbsp. olive oil
- 1/2 bunch, fresh coriander, finely cut
- Salt and pepper, to taste
- /2 cup heavy cream

## Direction

1. Heat the olive oil in a large pot over medium heat and sauté the onions, carrots, garlic and chili pepper until tender.
2. Add 4-5 cups of water and bring to a boil.
3. Reduce heat to low and simmer for 30 minutes.

4. Transfer the soup to a blender or food processor and blend until smooth.
5. Return to the pot and continue cooking for a few more minutes.
6. Remove the soup from heat and stir in the cream.
7. Serve with coriander sprinkled over each serving. Enjoy!

# Mushroom, Barley and Lentil Soup

**Servings:** 4

**Ingredients and Quantity**

- 2 medium leeks, trimmed, halved, sliced
- 10 white mushrooms, sliced
- 3 garlic cloves, cut
- 2 bay leaves
- 2 cans tomatoes, chopped, undrained
- 3/4 cup red lentils
- 1/3 cup barley
- 3 tbsp. extra virgin olive oil
- 1 tsp. paprika
- 1 tsp. savory
- 1/2 tsp. cumin

**Direction**

1. Heat oil in a large saucepan over medium-high heat.
2. Sauté leeks and mushrooms for 3 to 4 minutes or until softened.
3. Add cumin, paprika, savory and tomatoes, lentils, barley and 5 cups cold water.
4. Season with salt and pepper.
5. Cover and bring to a boil. Reduce the heat to low.
6. Simmer for 35 to 40 minutes or until barley is tender. Serve and enjoy!

# *Creamy Wild Mushroom Soup*

**Servings:** 4

## Ingredients and Quantity

- 2 cups wild mushrooms, peeled and chopped
- 1 onion, chopped
- 2 garlic cloves, crushed and chopped
- 1 tsp. dried thyme
- 3 cups vegetable broth
- Salt and pepper, to taste
- 3 tbsp. olive oil

## Direction

1. Sauté onions and garlic in a large soup pot till transparent.
2. Add thyme and mushrooms.
3. Cook for 10 minutes then add the vegetable broth and simmer for another 10-20 minutes.
4. Blend, season and serve. Enjoy!

VEGETARIAN SALADS

# *Mediterranean Buckwheat Salad*

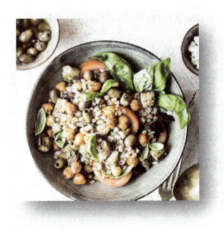

**Servings:** 4

**Ingredients and Quantity**

- 1 cup buckwheat grouts
- 1 3/4 cups water1 small red onion, finely chopped 1/2 cucumber, diced
- 1 cup cherry tomatoes, halved
- 1 yellow bell pepper, chopped
- A bunch parsley, finely cut

- 1 preserved lemon, finely chopped
- cup chickpeas, cooked or canned, drained Juice of half lemon
- 1 tsp. dried basil
- 2 tbsp. extra virgin olive oil
- Salt and black pepper, to taste

**Direction**

1. Heat a large, dry saucepan and toast the buckwheat for about 3 minutes.
2. Boil the water and add it carefully to the buckwheat.
3. Cover, reduce heat and simmer until buckwheat is tender and all liquid is absorbed (5-7 minutes).
4. Remove from heat, fluff with a fork and set aside to cool.
5. Mix the buckwheat with the chopped onion, bell pepper, cucumber, cherry tomatoes, parsley, preserved lemon and chickpeas in a salad bowl.
6. Whisk the lemon juice, olive oil and basil, season with salt and pepper to taste, then pour over the salad and stir.
7. Serve at room temperature. Enjoy!

# Beet and Bean Sprout Salad

**Servings:** 4

**Ingredients and Quantity**

- 7 beet greens, finely sliced
- 2 medium tomatoes, sliced
- 1 cup bean sprouts, washed
- 2 garlic cloves, crushed
- 1/2 cup each for lemon juice, olive oil
- 1 tsp. salt

**Direction**

1. In a large bowl, toss together beet greens, bean sprouts, tomatoes, and dressing.
2. Mix oil and lemon juice with lemon rind, salt and garlic and pour over the salad.
3. Refrigerate for 2 hours to allow flavor to develop before serving.
4. Best served chilled. Enjoy!

# *Tasty Tabbouleh*

**Servings:** 6

**Ingredients and Quantity**

- 1 cup raw bulgur
- 2 cups boiling water
- A bunch of parsley, finely cut
- 2 tomatoes, finely cut
- 2 tomatoes, chopped
- 3 tbsp. olive oil
- 2 garlic cloves, minced
- 6 to 7 fresh green onions, chopped
- 1 tbsp. fresh mint leaves, chopped
- Juice of 2 lemons
- Salt and black pepper, to taste

**Direction**

1. Bring water and salt to a boil, and then pour over bulgur.
2. Cover and set aside for 15 minutes to steam.
3. Drain excess water from bulgur and fluff with a fork. Leave it to chill.

4. In a large bowl, mix together the parsley, tomatoes, olive oil, garlic, green onions and mint.
5. Stir in the chilled bulgur and season to taste with salt, pepper and lemon juice. Serve and enjoy!

# *Savory Fatoush*

**Servings:** 6

**Ingredients and Quantity**

- 2 cups lettuce, washed, dried and chopped
- 3 tomatoes, chopped
- 1 cucumber, peeled and chopped
- 1 green pepper, seeded and chopped
- 1/2 cup radishes, sliced in half
- 1 small red onion, finely chopped
- 1/2 bunch parsley, finely cut
- 2 tbsp. fresh mint, finely chopped
- 3 tbsp. extra virgin olive oil
- 4 tbsp. lemon juice
- Salt and black pepper, to taste
- 2 whole-wheat pita breads

**Direction**

1. Toast the pita breads in a skillet until they are browned and crispy. Then set aside.
2. Place the lettuce, tomatoes, cucumbers, green pepper, radishes, onion, parsley and mint in a salad bowl.
3. Break up the toasted pita into bite-size pieces and add to the salad.
4. Make the dressing by whisking together the olive oil with the lemon juice, a pinch of salt and some black pepper.
5. Toss everything together until vegetables are well coated with the dressing. Serve and enjoy!

# *Chickpea Salad (Greek Style)*

**Servings:** 4

**Ingredients and Quantity**

- 1 cup canned chickpeas, drained and rinsed
- 1 spring onion, thinly sliced
- 1 small cucumber, deseeded and diced
- 2 green bell peppers, diced
- 2 tomatoes, diced
- 2 tsp. fresh parsley, chopped
- 1 tsp. capers, drained and rinsed
- Juice of 1/2 lemon
- 2 tbsp. extra virgin olive oil
- 1 tsp. balsamic vinegar
- Salt and pepper, to taste
- A pinch dried oregano

**Direction**

1. In a medium bowl, toss together the chickpeas, spring onion, cucumber, bell pepper, tomato, parsley, capers and lemon juice.
2. In a smaller bowl, stir together the remaining ingredients and pour over the chickpea salad.
3. Toss well to coat and allow to marinate, stirring occasionally, for at least one hour before serving. Enjoy!

# Red Cabbage Salad

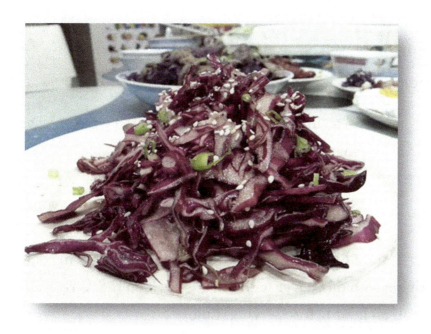

**Servings:** 6

**Ingredients and Quantity**

- 1 small head red cabbage, cored and chopped
- 1 bunch fresh dill, finely cut
- 3 tbsp. sunflower oil
- 3 tbsp. red wine vinegar
- 1 tsp. Sugar

- 2 tsp. salt
- Black pepper, to taste

## Direction

1. In a cup, mix the sunflower oil, red wine vinegar, sugar and black pepper.
2. Place the cabbage in a large glass bowl.
3. Sprinkle the salt on top and crunch it with your hands to soften.
4. Pour dressing over the cabbage and toss to coat.

Sprinkle with dill, cover with foil and leave in the refrigerator for half an hour before serving. Enjoy!

www.ingramcontent.com/pod-product-compliance
Lightning Source LLC
LaVergne TN
LVHW020346140325
805954LV00008B/470